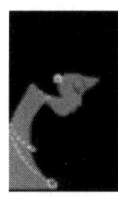

Sweet Melody Media
Publishing, Inc.

## Other Personal Care & Healthy Living Guides by this Author

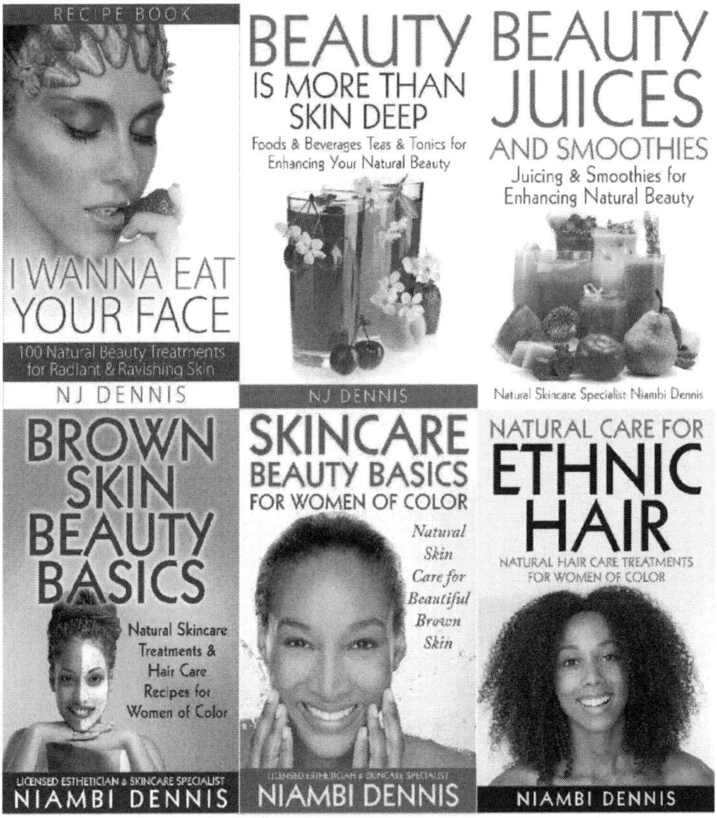

# SKINCARE BEAUTY BASICS FOR WOMEN OF COLOR

## Natural Skin Care
### *for Beautiful Brown Skin*

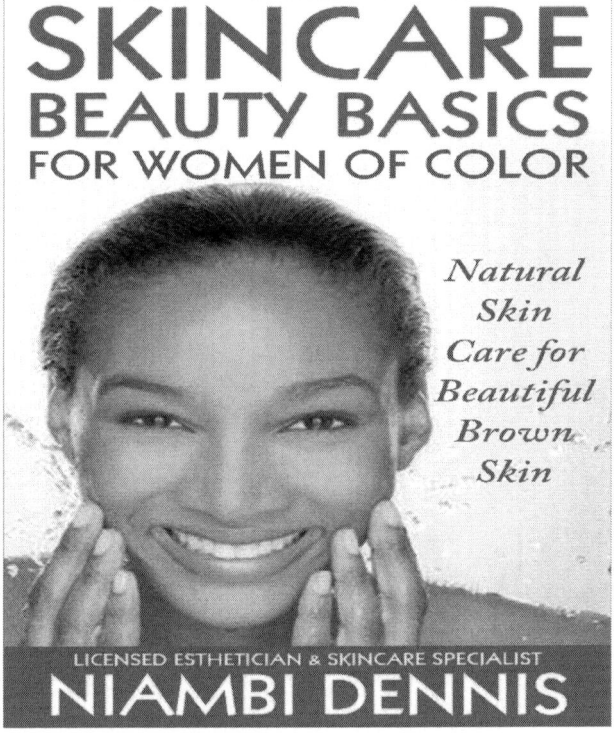

By **LICENSED ESTHETICIAN & NATURAL SKINCARE SPECIALIST**

*Niambi J Dennis*

Published by:

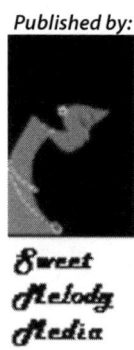

*Sweet
Melody
Media*

© Sweet Melody Media Publishing, Inc. 2015.
All rights reserved.

**SECOND EDITION COPYRIGHT ©2015**
Protected by copyright laws of the United States and international treaties.
No part of this publication may be copied, duplicated or reproduced in any form,
without the express written permission from the publisher.

Published and distributed globally thru: Sweet Melody Media Publishing

All rights reserved. No part of this book may be reproduced by any mechanical, photographic, or electronic process, or in the form of phonographic reading; nor may it be stored in a retrieval system, transmitted, or otherwise be copied for public or private use – other than for "fair use" as brief quotations embodied in articles and reviews – without written permission of the publisher.

The author of this book does not dispense medical advice or prescribe the use of any techniques as a form of treatment for physical, emotional, or medical problems without the advice of a physician, either directly or indirectly. The intent of the author is only to offer information of a general nature to help you in your quest for healthier living and balanced well-being. In the event that you use the information in this book for yourself, which is your constitutional right, the author and publisher assume no responsibility for your actions and or results thereof.

Printed in the USA

**ISBN-13:** 978-1517198268
**ISBN-10:** 1517198267

# *Forward*

In Sweet Remembrance of My Pop
Love You to Heaven and Back...

\*\*\*\*\*\*\*\*\*

### *A Love Note to All My Beautiful Brown Skin Sisters,*

You are comprised of sienna, chestnut and warm mahogany.
Dark as the night sky, constellations are tucked beneath your bones.
Your skin is reminiscent of hot chocolate that warms the soul.
Like rings around a tree, you too have history etched into your melanin.
Stand Tall My Sister, in Your Natural Black Beauty.

# TABLE OF CONTENTS

**NATURAL SKIN CARE INTRODUCTION**     **13**

  *Let's Get to It – Your Basic Routine*     *21*

  *First Step...We Cleanse* (Why & With What)     *23*

    In the Morning     23

    At Night     23

    My #1 Favorite Cleanser     24

  *Next We Tone* (Why & With What)     *27*

    Recipes for Homemade Facial Toners     31

  *Then We Moisturize* (Why & With What)     *35*

    Other One Ingredient Moisturizers     37

  *Exfoliating* (Why and With What)     *39*

    Good Exfoliating Options     42

  *Masking* (Why & With What)     *49*

    Powerful & Potent Masking Recipes     55

  *Natural Skin Care Conclusion*     *61*

**About the Author**     *63*

**Other Books by This Author**     *65*

**One More Thing**     *69*

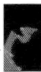

## NATURAL SKIN CARE INTRODUCTION

As Women of Color, we are blessed with the most BEAUTIFUL skin! Not only does it naturally glow, glisten and shine, it also gives us extra protection from the elements and even aging. With that being said, we must still take care of what God and Mother Nature have been so generous with. Besides, even good can get BETTER!

I'm a Licensed Esthetician currently specializing in Natural Skincare for Women of Color. For the last 3 years, 90% of the clients I see in my treatment room are Black and Brown. Usually the skin issues I see are easily treatable with common natural products, the client already has on hand.

After successfully treating and maintaining skin health for myself and my clients, I decided to put together this little guide to reach more women in need. The skincare element of this book will provide a foundation for your new healthy, glowing skin. It's easy to follow and perfect to build on.

For more comprehensive recipes for cleansing, toning, moisturizing and masking, all skin types, order a copy of *"I Wanna Eat Your Face"*, with over 100 beauty treatments.

For enhancing your natural beauty from the inside out, take a look at *"Beauty Is More than Skin Deep"*. Literally eat and drink your way to enhanced beauty. Learn which foods to load up on to increase healthy clear skin, make your hair grow like crazy and even help you get a better night's sleep!

**Cultivate your natural beauty by BEING beautiful and you will naturally LOOK more beautiful!**

## ~ *Before We Get Started* ~

Having clear healthy skin is easier than most people realize. All you need are the appropriate products for your skin, the proper techniques for application and a consistent regiment. People experience skin issues either because they are using the wrong products for their skin, they are using those products incorrectly, or they are not using them regularly. To be honest, it's usually a combination of all 3.

Usually, your skin suffers at your own hand. Unknowingly, we exacerbate our skin issues by the products we purchase. Many of these products strip off essential protective oils by using harsh chemicals. All-natural remedies do a fantastic job of cleaning your delicate facial skin, without harmful stripping. Not only do they remove dead skin cells and excess oils, but these cleansers will also dissolve dirt and other impurities, while providing rich nourishment.

Developing a highly customized beauty regiment, that's natural, potent and way under budget is very doable these days. **Keep reading to find out how!**

**A sound complete skincare regiment includes:**

Twice Daily Cleansing

Twice Daily Toning

Twice Daily Moisturizing

Twice Daily Eye Cream

Weekly Exfoliating

Weekly/Bi-Weekly Masking

**DON'T FORGET THE SUNSCREEN:** Now even though our skin is rich in melanin and we have a measure of protection, it is still very important that even Women of Color use sunscreen to protect ourselves from harmful ultra-violet rays. This will also help to slow down the effects of aging….even more!

There are a several factors that will impact your skin outside of what you put on it. Namely, what you put **IN** it! As much as possible, incorporate the following into your **Daily Beauty Regiment**:

- **Water:** Sufficient water intake is crucial to healthy clear skin. Drinking lots of water will keep your skin plump and hydrated, supple and glowing. It will also flush your pores and help them purge excess oils and other toxins. Not drinking enough water could cause excess dryness or oiliness, dull skin and sunken hollows. Not to mention **chronic acne**! At least 96oz. of water a day is ideal.

- **Fresh LIVE Foods:** Eating LIVE food will impart invaluable vitamins and nutrients into your skin's cell structure. Feeding your body a healthy, live, fresh, balanced diet, will also feed your skin all the goodness it needs to thrive! The foods you eat affect the tone and texture of your skin. **Eat pretty!**

- **Eat EXTRA GREENS:** Along with your LIVE Fresh Foods, you'll want to concentrate on eating lots of leafy greens. These are **full** of folic acid and iron, which will keep your skin looking fresh and clear, not to mention **make your hair grow like crazy**!!! Kale and spinach are especially good for beauty!

- **Adequate Sleep:** 8 – 10 hours is optimal Beauty Sleep is real...get yours! Not only does inadequate sleep create sallow, sullen skin, but it will prematurely age you. This gives a whole new meaning to the phrase *'sleep pretty'*!

- **Minimize Stress:** Overtime, stress will age you terribly. If you want to end up with a face full of wrinkles, cracks and crevices, continue to worry and stress!

    Learn not to sweat the small stuff, not to take things personally and to keep the main thing the main thing. Have faith in all optimal outcomes and release what no longer serves you. **You got this Girl Friend!**

Incorporating these activities into your daily routine will enhance your beauty quotient exponentially.

**Prime & protect your skin from the inside out!**

## Cleansing Tips

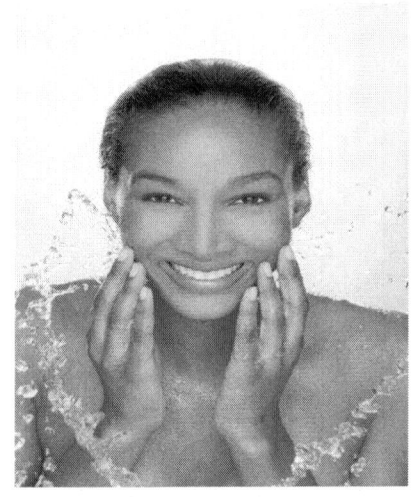

To maximize the benefits of your natural cleansers, always apply your recipes with damp hands, or to warm moist skin. You can even take a hot shower or a steam bath to open your pores, prior to cleansing. This will **prime** your skin and allow your ingredients to **penetrate deeper** into your epidermis.

Use small circular motions to gently massage your cleansers into your skin. Gently pat away excess moisture, or better yet, air dry, but whatever you do **never** wipe. Over time, wiping stretches delicate facial tissue, which leads to sagging & wrinkles. **So always gently pat to dry or just allow your skin to air dry!**

### A Note about Natural Facial Cleansers

Natural cleansers do not typically 'foam' or include foaming agents. Foaming is usually associated with retail products that contain harsh and unnecessary chemicals. While most home-made facial cleansers don't foam like retail cleansers, they also don't dry and damage the skin like traditional cleansers. Foaming agents are the #1 cause of drying, stripping and upsetting the pH balance of skin and hair. **Try to avoid these agents as much as possible**!

# ~ *Let's Get to It – Your Basic Routine* ~

It's best to develop a routine to really see and sustain healthy clear skin. Once you do it a few times it will become quick and easy and eventually second nature. Just get in the habit of doing what you need to do to achieve the results you're looking for.

**It's as easy as 1, 2, 3….4!**

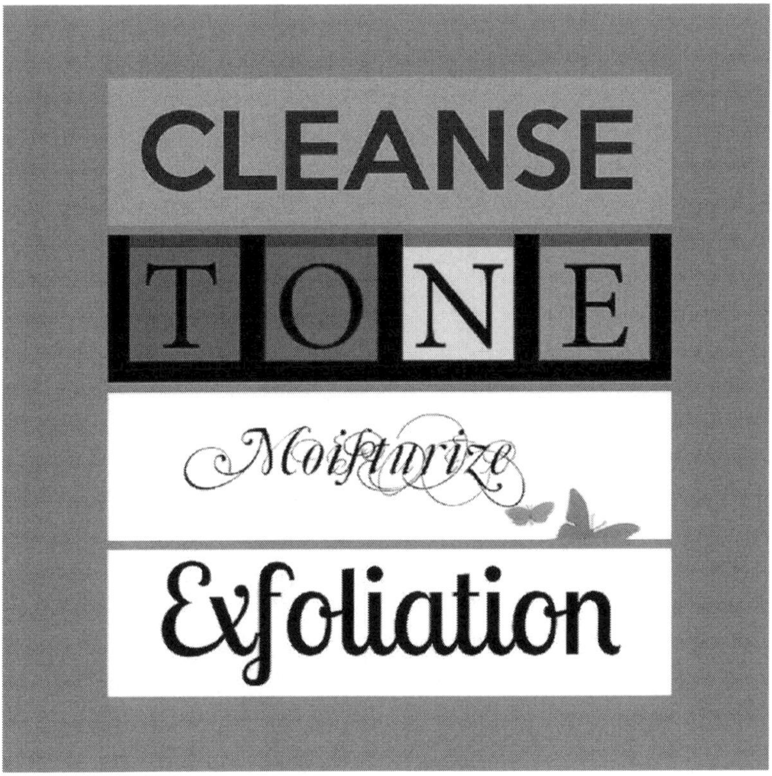

CLEANSE

TONE

Moisturize

Exfoliation

# ~ *First Step...We Cleanse* (*Why & With What*) ~

For best results, cleanse your skin at least twice a day. First thing in the morning and last thing in the evening. When you first wake up and just before you go to bed for the night.

## In the Morning

While you sleep, your pores open up and expel toxins and excess sebum (oil). About 10 minutes after you're up and moving around, your pores will close up and shut down. If you don't cleanse your skin adequately and quickly enough, your pores will reabsorb those toxins when they shut down, trapping and clogging them with dirty oil. This is a recipe for acne disaster!

## At Night

Your skin is a living, breathing organ. It's like a sponge; very porous and full of your environment. It will really absorb the smog, smoke, sweat, grease, sneezes, kisses, germs and bacteria you expose it to. The LAST thing you want to do is go to sleep in that nasty germy cesspool!

Again, your pores will relax overnight. If your face is covered with toxic soup, your pores will drink it up and deliver it to the deepest layers of your skin (dermis and subcutaneous layers), while you sleep! Then your pores will be sick in the morning! Keep your pores healthy by removing the day's environment from the surface of your skin and adding healthy night serums or moisturizing skin cocktails, before bedtime.

## My #1 Favorite Cleanser

My favorite facial cleanser is HONEY! Yep....HONEY! Regular honey that you would eat! Just plain ole honey.

Just squirt about the same amount into your wet hand that you would your regular cleanser, emulsify and apply to your skin in small circular motions. NOTE: Honey looses it's stickiness when it gets wet.

Gently massage. Rinse clear with **lukewarm to cool** water.

**Re-apply and repeat, as cleansing twice is most ideal.** Gently massage into damp skin. Rinse clear with **cool to cold** water. Get ready to tone.

**NOTE:** A general rule of thumb is to cleanse with warm water initially and do your final rinsing with cool or cold water. The warm water will open your pores and the cool water will close them down.

Plain honey makes a perfect natural cleanser for ALL skin types. Whether your skin is normal, oily, dry, acneic, aging or anything in between, honey can literally heal your skin and most skin conditions.

Honey is anti-microbial and anti-bacterial. It's a natural humectant, which will gently hydrate your skin without any extra oiliness. It dissolves excess sebum (oil) and feeds your pores rich natural nutrients. It will naturally regulate the pH level of your skin and keep it balanced and happy.

You will see results after the first uses, but will really reap the benefits with continued regular usage. The cumulative effect of consistent honey usage on your skin is healthy, clear, glowing skin.

Using honey won't guarantee that you'll never get another break-out, but it will minimize the frequency of future break-outs and reduce the duration of any existing inflammation.

Before I started using honey about 7 years ago, I had what most would consider 'problem skin'. It was overly oily, acne prone and very temperamental. Since honey has been a regular staple in my skincare program, I rarely have any skin issues at all. My skin is not just clear, but balanced and healthy. Much of this is due to my consistent usage of the nectar of the gods, which I regularly use in cleansing, exfoliating and masking.

## ~ *Next We Tone* *(Why & With What)* ~

Toning is an integral component in your healthy skin regiment. A good toner is a multi-purpose tool for skin health and beauty. Not only will a toner remove any trace elements of cleanser you may have left behind, but a good one will also restore the optimal pH balance to your skin. Toning primes your skin nicely for a moisturizing sealer.

Toning is a very important step that many often overlook. Most skin issues arise from an imbalance in your skin's physiology. They can also be caused by an imbalance in your body's physiology. So either outside or inside, if you have chronic skin issues, you are out of balance Dear Heart.

Very good, stand alone, toner options are:
- aloe juice
- rose water
- witch hazel
- diluted apple cider vinegar
- a little diluted vodka
- even fresh juiced ginger or cucumber

All of these are great options for healing, soothing, hydrating and imparting a dewy glow to your skin. These "stand-alone" ingredients are also great to add to your more complex recipes.

Toning with natural, products will help to restore and or maintain optimal balance for your skin. I make my own toning solution and just keep it in a small 12 oz. bottle in my medicine cabinet. Usually my toners are Aloe Vera juice based; again, chosen because of its natural healing and pH balancing properties.

Very often, I mix in a little booster of Tea Tree Oil with my Aloe Vera juice based toner.

**Tea Tree Oil:** Tea Tree Oil is great for your skin! If you have particularly oily or acne prone skin, I would strongly suggest you start incorporating Tea Tree Oil into your skin care regiment slowly.

It will help to combat the growth of any bacteria that may be brewing on the surface or even at deeper layers of your skin. Tea Tree Oil will not only treat and minimize existing acne issues, but can stop future outbreaks before they even get started, or at least decrease the length of time and severity that they present.

It's very strong, so you only need to mix a few drops in with your aloe juice, witch hazel, green tea, or diluted vodka to create a fantastic and budget friendly toner. Play around with your ideal proportions. **You will only need a couple, few drops for about 24oz. of toner.**

**Bamboo Extract** is another fantastic toning booster, I love to include in my skincare program.

Yep, I'm talking bamboo, like from the tree! The silica in Bamboo will help stimulate cell turnover in the epidermis (top few layers) of your skin. Increased cell turnover means that your skin is creating more new healthy cells and shedding the older, duller, lack luster cells faster. The results are the appearance of clearer, healthier skin. I order my Bamboo extract from Amazon.

Bamboo Extract is tremendous for stimulating and accelerating hair growth as well! ☺

Just shake your mixtures well, before each use. Lightly moisten a cotton round or cotton square and gently dab your toner all over face and neck after cleansing. I don't even dry my face after the cleanse, I just grab a cotton round, saturate it and wipe my face and neck down.

## Recipes for Homemade Facial Toners

If you'd like to customize your toner even more, here are a few recipes for you to choose from. Pick the ones that address your specific needs and preferences.

**Easy Green Tea Toner:** This is a favorite of mine. It's super simple and leaves your skin glowing and toned. Gently boil (on low) a bag of your favorite Green Tea (look for those that are high in anti-oxidants) in 2 – 3 cups of water. Allow your tea bag to steep for 15 minutes to a half an hour. This is a great time to make a fresh scrub and exfoliate your face! You can also use the steam to give yourself a soothing treatment. Once done remove your tea bags and allow tea to cool. You can either use your Green Tea Toner as is or dilute/stretch it with 1 – 2 cups more water, or even better, Aloe Vera Juice.

You can also add 1 – 2 Tbsp of honey for increased hydration, up to 5 drops of tea tree oil to reduce bacteria growth, or a splash of Vodka to increase the astringent qualities of your toner.

**Chamomile Toner:** If you have inflamed, irritated, problematic or very sensitive skin, chamomile tea makes a great choice for a very mild healing toner. Steep your tea bag or loose tea in a cup or more of water for at least 5 minutes. Apply with cotton round. No need to rinse or refrigerate.

**Sweet Apple-Tini Toner**

The vodka in this one makes it a more astringent. If you're looking for a stronger toner, use this one. Blend together 1 tablespoon honey, 1 tablespoon of vodka, ½-1 cup of water or aloe juice and one peeled, cored apple. Apply this refreshing mixture and allow it to sit for at least 15 minutes. Go have a conversation with someone you love. Tell them how much you love them!

Once you're done, rinse your face clear with lukewarm water.

**Apple Tart Toner**

This powerful toner is an excellent choice for oily skin. Witch Hazel and ACV are gentle astringents that will help restore your skin's natural pH balance, while lavender soothes sensitive skin.

Ingredients:

- ⅔ cup of Witch Hazel
- ⅓ cup of Apple Cider Vinegar
- Several drops of Lavender Oil (or Essential Oil of your choice)

Mix ingredients thoroughly in a clean bottle. Shake vigorously before each use. Dampen a cotton round with toner and gently wipe across face. Can be stored at room temperature.

**Just a note:** Most Sisters of Color that I see in my treatment room complain of oily skin. Many will try to combat and "dry up" this oiliness with alcohol based toners and even worse, isopropyl alcohol ITSLEF! BIG NO-NO! I repeat…..DO NOT DO THIS! This will only make a bad situation much, much worse!

By stripping your skin and temporarily drying out your pores with harsh alcohol, you are basically programming your pores to go into over-drive producing excess oil and sebum. It's a biological, physiological chain reaction that you have set into motion.

If you use alcohol on your face, get ready for an oil slick in... **3-2-1**!!!

Just don't ever do it!! You're making the problem so much worse. The most important factor in your skin health is balance. Isopropyl alcohol will throw your skin totally out of balance and it will never naturally recover! Your pores will be in a perpetual state of shock and hyper activity.

So check the ingredients in your retail products and steer very clear of any products with even a drop of alcohol. You and your skin will thank me later!

Have fun making these dynamite toners and get ready to fall in love with your clear fresh skin.

Ahhhh....now your skin is nice and fresh and ready to receive your moisturizer.

## ~ *Then We Moisturize* (Why & With What) ~

The biggest mistake most of the Sisters I see in my treatment room make is NOT moisturizing at all! 8 out of 10 Women of Color feel they have oily skin or would describe their skin as oily. In an effort to combat this oiliness, they make the cardinal mistake of skipping the moisturizer! This actually creates and increases the very issue she's trying to avoid!

The key is to moisturize without any added oiliness or greasy residue.

**My #1 natural daytime moisturizer is Aloe Vera gel.** Aloe gel is calming, balancing and healing. You can purchase a pre-packaged 100% gel, or you can harvest it straight from the plant if you have access to live Aloe Vera. If you are purchasing retail, make sure you opt for a brand that is clear, not blue or green, as these contain not only unnatural dyes, but usually alcohol, as well.

Once you've toned with the natural toner of your choice, squirt a small amount of Aloe gel into your damp hand and gently apply it to your skin. Allow it to naturally absorb and air dry. This will act as a serum that imparts moisture, without any residue or greasy filmy feeling. Once it totally dries, your face will feel fresher and even a bit tighter.

Even in my mid-forties, I usually go out bare faced, because my skin can stand alone and even shines on its own! My cleansing, toning and moisturizing regiment is the reason why.

## Other One Ingredient Moisturizers

**Oil** has been used as a moisturizer long before actual moisturizing products were sold. Olive or even Grape seed oil hydrate, soothe and heal skin. These 'heavier' moisturizers work best for night-time treatments, as they may be a bit too heavy for daytime usage. However, they will mix nicely with other lighter ingredients. A little goes a long way. **Oils work well for night-time nourishing.**

**Coconut Oil** is divine for all skin types. It's not as "oily" as say an Olive or Grape Seed Oil and it absorbs like a dream into your skin. As with all oil applications, a little goes a long way. Coconut oil is a great sealer and locks moisture into your skin and hair.

**Shea Butter** is one of my favorite skin and hair moisturizers. You'll find that 100% Shea Butter is very dense and hard. I like to gently heat it until it's soft in a double boiler. I mix in a couple tablespoons of coconut oil to soften it up and make it easier to apply. You can also add some of your favorite Essential Oils at this time. I pour my liquid mixture into small plastic air-tight containers. Allow your moisturizer to sit for a couple/few days until it re-congeals and forms a light dense cream. This moisturizer makes my skin really radiant, especially when I apply it at night. It's a great night-time eye treatment. Shea Butter won't clog your pores and instead nourishes your skin at deeper levels. My hair also loves it!

**Emu Oil** is a fantastic light moisturizing oil. It works great alone and also works well mixed in with heavier carrying creams. The molecules in this oil are very small, allowing it to penetrate your epidermis and reach your dermis. This oil heals and feeds your skin from the inside out. It makes a great anti-aging component and is also great for healing break-outs.

***Vitamin E** makes a great addition to just about any skin or body treatment. Consider adding a few drops or drizzles into your recipes and concoctions. Vitamin E is great for correcting blemishes and discolorations. It will even soothe and heal your cracked cuticles and lips. It's also helpful for eyelash growth. It's also light enough to be used as a daytime moisturizer for your eye area.

NOTE: When applying to your face, use the tiniest amounts to start. Only add more if needed. You will soon learn the perfect amount for you. Apply your moisturizers to damp skin, after properly cleansing and toning.

## ~ *Exfoliating* *(Why and With What)* ~

What is exfoliating and why do you need to do it regularly?

Exfoliating is simply the process of removing dead skin cells from the skin's epidermis or outer surface layer. Removing this dead skin makes way for the younger skin cells underneath. Dry, dead skin cells clog your pores, leading to blackheads, acne and many other problems. When dead skin is removed, beautiful, more luminous skin is revealed. Regular exfoliation can also help reduce blotchiness, sun-damage and discoloration. Exfoliating on a consistent basis is critical to your skin's health and radiance.

By gently exfoliating away the top layer of dead cells, your skin will feel smoother, look more vibrant and age slower. Just the act of rubbing in a circular motion, increases circulation and improves your overall health. While the exfoliating agent carries away that top layer of dull cells.

Think of it as buffing your skin out. Not so much scrubbing, but more gentle buffing and refining.

Many Sisters will use 'scrubs' in an effort to scrape out and scrape off excess oil. Guess what...using harsh, overly abrasive products or even exfoliating too often will do more harm than good.

**Two Things:**

1. That **Apricot Scrub** (I won't mention the brand, but we ALL know it!) is the **ABSOLUTE WORST**! The apricot pits are ground in with this pasty, goopy mixture, but usually not very well. These pit particles are too large, sharp and abrasive for delicate facial skin. This scrub will actually make a skin issue much worse, because it will open up small surface nicks on the surface of your skin. I can tell clients who use this without even asking. As soon as I get them under my magnifying lamp, I can clearly see tiny scrapes and cuts all along the skin's surface.

Not only does this damage your epidermis, but it opens up areas in the skin for cross contamination. So that bacteria in the zit that's on your chin, is transferred and migrates to your forehead, cheeks, nose, etc. etc. etc. Creating a full-blown acne outbreak!

In addition to all the sharp pit particles, this particular apricot scrub is full of harsh chemicals, fillers and preservatives that are not good for your skin. **DO NOT USE THIS STUFF!**

**2. Avoid OVER-Exfoliating.** When I do my initial consultations, many of my clients state that they actually exfoliate EVERYDAY!!! **This is a BIG No-No!**

When my Little Sister revealed to me that she actually exfoliated with that doggone Apricot Scrub…. DAILY!!!! I nearly fell out of my chair! LITERALLY! I instantly thought to myself, "No WONDER your skin looks like THAT!"

That stuff is HORRIBLE for your skin, most especially your facial skin…and every day???? Please…Knock it OFF Ma'am!

Avoid the MISTAKE of over-exfoliating; which can either be done with the exfoliating products, methods of exfoliating or frequency of exfoliating.

Exfoliating with harsh and harmful products can compromise your epidermis (the top layer of your skin). Scrubbing or abrading too harshly can cause damage to your delicate facial skin. Avoid pressing too hard as you can easily scratch, knick and/or cut the surface layers of your skin.

Even when using appropriate products and pressure, you can still adversely affect your skin by exfoliating too frequently. You never exfoliate more than two or three times per week. Typically, once a week or twice a month is sufficient for normal healthy skin.

Exfoliating too often will cause microscopic tears, which will lead to premature aging, wrinkles and sallowness. It will also cause your skin to produce excess oil and enlarge your pores. None of which you want!!!

If you use Exfoliation wisely in your Skincare Program, your skin will be glowing in no time!

## Good Exfoliating Options

**Cinnamon:** One of my favorite granular exfoliating agents is cinnamon. It improves overall circulation and gives your scrubs an exhilarating scent. It is very healing and effective for calming break-outs and inflammation. Cinnamon is great to incorporate into your facial applications.

**My #1 Go-To Quick & EZ Exfoliator** is honey with a sprinkle of cinnamon. Easy and very effective skin buffer. Just moisten your hand. Add a small shot of honey. Add a sprinkle of cinnamon on top. Emulsify (rub your hands together). Gently apply in small circular motions to your skin. Can rinse immediately, or leave to sit for several minutes. It may tingle, especially if you leave it on. This is normal.

Rinse very **very** good. Finish with another honey cleanse (honey only). You will probably feel cinnamon residue in your eyelashes and possibly around your face perimeter. Cleanse and rinse all this away and follow up with a good toner.

**Baking Soda:** Baking Soda is a nice extra gentle buffer. It's much more gentle and less abrasive than a sugar, salt or coffee scrub. You can incorporate a baking soda component in to a simple honey wash several times per week to gently buff your complexion clear.

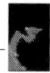

Baking Soda is even very effective for minimizing pores and resurfacing skin. Make sure you rinse clean and clear. And because baking soda has such a low pH, you'll want to make sure you follow with a pH balancing toner. Aloe Vera Juice or even a diluted acidic solution (lemon juice, apple cider vinegar, for example) will work nicely. Finish with an appropriate moisturizer for your skin.

**Niacin Powder:** Niacin masks can be over $100 in the treatment room. Niacin is very effective at reducing pore size and stimulating cell turnover. It also is very powerful at helping other vitamins and nutrients applied topically to penetrate more deeply. Niacin helps to restore your skins natural self-healing mechanism. It also creates a barrier that helps to correct and combat the signs of aging.

Exfoliating regularly with Niacin helps to enable healing and to improve skin tone and texture, repair damage, and build a natural barrier for the skin. To use, just break open 1 Niacin capsule and sprinkle the powder in your hand. You'll need a carrying agent, such as honey (I know...my favorite), your favorite retail product will work as well, if you prefer. Emulsify the powder and carrier together and apply to your skin. Either rinse immediately or leave to sit. Rinse well. Finish with toning and moisturizing.

**Turmeric Powder:** I've saved one of the best for last! Turmeric is naturally antiseptic, anti-inflammatory and anti-microbial. There are so many benefits from using this powerful spice topically, I lose count sometimes.

**Some things Turmeric can be helpful for:**

**Healthy Glowing Skin:** When I exfoliate my face with turmeric it shines bright like a diamond! Seriously, using turmeric as an exfoliating agent will brighten your skin tone and really make you look like you're glowing. After using turmeric for just a short time, it will look like you have a flashlight following you around! To optimize your skin's health, exfoliate with turmeric once or twice a week.

You can mix your turmeric down with honey, milk, aloe juice, water, and many other gentle carriers. For exfoliating, you'll want to be heavier on the carrier. For example, if you are using water, you are not looking to make a paste, as you would for a masking application. To exfoliate, you want to be able to easily and smoothly abrade the skin's surface without too much friction. So, in general, thinner is a better consistency for the exfoliating application.

Gently apply the loose mixture to your face in small circular motions. Give yourself a light massage; always taking care to work in gentle upward motions. Rinse **thoroughly**, with warm to cool water. Make sure you do a follow-up cleanse, or two, (**rinsing with COLD water**) to remove any granules of spice left behind. *Finish with toning and moisturizing.*

**Anti-Aging:** Turmeric is also a great anti-oxidant that helps fend off free-radicals, which age your skin prematurely. Consistently using turmeric as an exfoliating agent will reduce signs of aging. Apply in the same manner as above.

**Acne Relief:** Turmeric will even help calm and shorten the duration of any active acne break-outs. If your face is erupting, calm it down by exfoliating with a turmeric and milk 'scrub'. This will reduce excess oil secretion from the sebaceous glands and naturally reduce inflammation. Since turmeric is also antiseptic and anti-microbial, it will also help to heal the bacterial out break that's present in your acneic pores.

**Powerful Pimple Pucker:** add some lemon juice and water to turmeric powder to form a loose consistency. Gently exfoliate. Take care not to 'scrub' too hard over active acne. Let the treatment do the work! For severe cases of acne, allow this exfoliating mask to set up for 10 or 15 minutes. Remoisten with warm water and gently rinse away. Cleanse again. Tone and Moisturize.

**Acne Scars/ Dark Spots/ Discoloration/ Hyperpigmentation:** Over time, turmeric will help normalize uneven skin tone. Many of my clients say that they were able to stop wearing foundation after regularly using turmeric on their skin. To reduce acne scars, apply a mixture of turmeric powder and lemon juice or cucumber on acne marks and leave on for up to 15 minutes. This will significantly **reduce pigmentation** and even out your skin tone.

**Stretch Marks:** Turmeric has been used for many centuries to prevent and reduce the appearance of stretch marks. During pregnancy women would regularly treat their bellies and thighs with pastes and potions rich in turmeric to reduce the appearance of skin stretching.

Avoid stretch marks before they even get started or minimize what's already there by applying a mixture of turmeric and yogurt to your affected areas. Leave it for about 5 minutes, then rinse clear. If you continue this regularly, it will **help in maintaining the elasticity of your skin and make your virtually stretch marks proof!**

**Healing Burns:** If you're a little bit of a klutz, like me, then you will love turmeric for it's ability to soothe and heal minor burns. It's antiseptic properties will help with stinging, swelling and healing the affected area in no time. Plus you have the added benefit of turmeric's natural ability to combat skin discoloration. For minor skin burns, mix turmeric powder with Aloe Vera gel and apply on affected area.

*Extra Luxurious Pamper Days:* Exfoliate with a paste of dissolved sugar syrup, buttermilk and turmeric powder. Make it into a paste and apply to face to reduce wrinkles **and** dark circles.

Use paste made from turmeric powder and honey paste to exfoliate skin and reduce pores.

**Oily Skin Mask:** Turmeric is a good treatment for oily skin, because it helps regulate the production of sebum, which is an oily substance produced by your sebaceous glands. Mixing it with a bit of orange juice will be powerful astringent for clearing out oily pores.

**Slowing Hair Growth:** If you're getting the Lady Mustache growing in and you don't want to wax, shave, tweeze or thread, you can slow down the actual rate of growth by using turmeric as an exfoliating agent and even mask on the areas of concern.

Do this treatment regularly for about a month to see best results. Like most natural treatments, you will see a cumulative effect with the consistent usage of this application.

**Quick & EZ:** For a quick, easy and extra powerful exfoliating treatment, I will put some turmeric, cinnamon and honey in my damp hand, emulsify and gently massage my face. This simple healing and fortifying exfoliator will gently buff out your skin and turn up your glow!

**A couple things to remember when using turmeric:**

1. Since turmeric can slow down hair growth, avoid your eyebrows and eyelashes as much as possible when exfoliating and masking with turmeric or recipes that include turmeric on the ingredient list.

2. Be careful, as it can temporarily stain your skin, depending on your complexion. Very light complected Sisters may see a bit of a yellow tinge left behind temporarily, this will subside shortly. Turmeric generally shows up on Browner/Darker skin tones as a lovely glow.

Can you tell I LOVE turmeric? I really do! It's versatile and so healing for all skin types. A great natural solution for any number of skin issues. Fantastic for general health and nutrition of your skin. Add it to your Skincare Program **today!**

## ~ *Masking* (Why & With What) ~

### *Mother Earth Skin Flourishes with Rich Earthy Treatments*

Masking your skin is the time when you get to nourish it and love on it a little bit extra! You mask your skin after a thorough and sometimes deep cleansing. Often times after a good exfoliating treatment. So your pores are open and ready to receive your vitamin packed masking treatment. Since your pores are primed and ready to receive, be selective about what you feed them.

You'll want to apply your mask with your fingers or a facial brush (or soft small paint brush). Choose the best tool for the masking paste you're using. After masking, you will want to follow-up with a quick cleanse, to remove any excess residue and particles. I use a simple honey cleanse, but you can use your favorite cleanser here. Always finish with a good toner and moisturizer.

Keep reading for some simple one or two ingredient treatments and a few more complex masking recipes. If you'd like more Beauty Mask Recipes for your eReader, be sure to download *"I Wanna Eat Your Face"*, for over 100 all natural skincare recipes for all skin types.

*So, to pick up where we left off...Turmeric.*

As you've probably figured out, if it makes a good exfoliator, it makes a great mask! For all the reasons you want to apply turmeric topically as an exfoliating agent, you'll also want to include it in your masking treatments, as well. Any of the exfoliating treatments using turmeric would also work nicely as masking treatments. Just make the consistency thicker and allow them to sit for several minutes (10-30) before rinsing.

For your masking treatments, you'll want the consistency to be much thicker. You are looking for a paste. Something that won't slide off and run down, while you're marinating. You want it thick, but not too thick. Ideally you want something you can spread in a nice, even, thin layer.

## *Neem Powder & Neem Oil Mask*

When I have a particularly stubborn pimple or area of inflammation and I'm not getting the results I'm looking for with my normal methods, I bring out the BIG GUNS! My potent and powerful Neem Mask! It's made from Neem powder, Neem oil, a little Rose water (all of which can be ordered online or found at your local Indian grocery food store) and a dash of Tea Tree Oil.

Neem is a fantastic natural astringent! It can be harsh, which is why I call it my BIG GUN, but if used sparingly, it can be very effective at keeping skin clear and free of break-outs, inflammation and excess oil. The Rose Water is hydrating and is great for balance in this mask. The Tea Tree Oil packs a powerful anti-microbial, anti-bacterial punch!

You mix everything up to make a paste. Not too loose, because you'll want it to sit for a while (anywhere from 10-30 minutes or so). During that time, why don't you go write a Love Letter to someone special...maybe it's YOU!

Once your face is done cooking, rinse very thoroughly. You're going to want to rinse extra and finish with a cleansing.

I use my honey. Just straight honey, but you can use your favorite cleanser here. Cleanse again thoroughly, making sure you get all the residue and particles out of your lashes and perimeter of your face, around your nose, etc. You'll have mask in interesting places!

Once you're clean and clear, **tone**, preferably with a natural toner. Rose water would work nicely here, due to it's hydrating properties. It will help counter-balance any drying from the astringent Neem powder. If you don't have Rose water, Aloe Vera juice is a good substitute. **After toning, moisturize!**

I recommend masking twice per month for normal skin. Once a week for treating problem issues. Neem products are great to add to your masks to boost their strength and corrective powers.

Just a note of caution....Neem Oil **stinks**! So don't say I didn't warn you!! :)

### *Bentonite Clay*

Bentonite clay is composed of ashes from volcanoes. This clay is very healing. So much so, it's affectionately called, *The Healing Clay*. Use it to detoxify and clear your skin of harmful poisons and bacteria.

Bentonite clay is known to have an abundance of minerals including calcium, magnesium, silica, sodium, copper, iron, and potassium, making it highly nourishing for your skin. It's even helpful for clearing eczema, psoriasis and dermatitis.

To mask with Bentonite, combine the clay with water. Apply liberally to skin and allow to dry. The clay will bind to any bacteria and toxins living on the surface of your skin **and** within your pores to extract the toxins.

This mask will help to reduce the break-outs, blemishes and alleviate redness. It also fights allergic reactions to irritating lotions or facial cleansers and even helps to soothe poison ivy.

Due to Bentonite Clay's ability to act as a topical antibiotic treatment, it can be helpful for calming skin infections and speeding up the healing time of minor cuts and wounds, even when prescription antibiotics have not been able to help solve the problem.

## Emu Oil

Emu Oil is original to the Aboriginal culture and has been used for centuries. Emu oil is rich in fatty acids, including Omega-3, Omega-6 and Omega-9. It is also non-comedogenic (which means it will **not** clog your pores). Used topically, it has numerous benefits for the skin.

Many moisturizers only work on the epidermis of your skin, which are the DEAD top outer layers. Because of the size of the molecules of most oils, they won't penetrate all the way down to the dermis, which are the LIVE layers underneath. Emu Oil has smaller molecules, which will make it to your fatty dermis layer, providing nourishment and protection at a deeper level.

Wrinkles and fine lines diminish, spots from aging can be reduced and healthy, new cells make your complexion look fresh and radiant. Your skin's elasticity will improve, as well as its clarity.

This oil is anti-microbial and anti-bacterial, so it is ideal for combating acne. Pimples are caused when bacteria gets clogged in your pores, which causes swelling and inflammation. The healing properties in Emu oil help eliminate bacteria in your skin, preventing break-outs and blemishes.

Generously add Emu Oil to your masking mixtures. Since it absorbs so quickly and completely, It even works great as a light stand alone moisturizer and night-time treatment. You can also mix a couple drops in with your favorite creamy moisturizer.

## Powerful & Potent Masking Recipes

Enjoy this free preview of *"I Wanna Eat Your Face"*.

The following facial mask recipes range from extra gentle for sensitive to normal skin, to more aggressive treatments for problematic skin.

*"I Wanna Eat Your Face"* has over 100 beauty recipes for naturally cleansing, toning, moisturizing, masking, and exfoliating. Plus you'll learn best skincare practices. If you're ready for more detailed recipes, DOWNLOAD it for your electronic reader at Amazon NOW!

**Let's start with a simple, but very powerful treatment!**

*Sunshine in a Bottle – Hydrating Tightening Mask*

You'll find that this recipe works beautifully for masking your skin! The ACV is clarifying in this recipe. The lemon juice will help even out your skin tone. Great mask for reducing the appearance of blemishes and acne scarrng.

*Ingredients:*

- 1 oz of Olive Oil
- 1 Egg
- 1 Tbsp of Lemon Juice
- 1 tsp of Apple Cider Vinegar

Churn ingredients in blender. Paint mixture on face in layered process. Once each layer dries, add another layer on top. Repeat this up to 3 times.

After final layer is dried, rinse thoroughly. Finish with toning and moisturizing.

## Hot Honey Masque

When it comes to dry skin, one of the best ingredients to use in your facial masks is honey. It not only works well as a cleanser, but also as a masque for creating radiant, healthy skin.

Place your bottle of honey in a sink full of hot water or even in lightly boiling water for a few minutes. You want the honey to get warm and glazy, but not cook or boil in any way.

I don't recommend the microwave, but obviously it's totally up to you. While your honey is warming, place a face cloth in hot water. Once it's very warm, wring out the excess water and apply to face. Hold in place for several seconds. Re-wet cloth with hot water and repeat. This will open your pores, allowing the nutrients in the honey to penetrate deeper.

**WHILE YOU'RE WAITING:** Apply your warmed honey to your face and go visualize your version of success for about 10–20 minutes. Think about what it means to and for you. Who will you impact? **What good will your success do others?**

When you're done, gently rinse with warm water, then with cold water to close your pores. As always, finish with a toner and moisturizer

This treatment reveals radiant, smooth, healthy-looking skin. Use this simple, but highly effective mask once or twice a week for maximum cumulative effects.

## Basic Bentonite Clay Facial Mask

This purifying mask will remove toxins and impurities from your pores. If your pores are large and clogged, this mask will help them purge. You will want to mask no more than once a week and at least once a month.

This basic clay mask will do a great job clarifying and calming inflamed skin. Soothe pimples and pustules by following this recipe. It's very forgiving and will accept many substitutions and additions.

### Ingredients:

- 2-3 oz of Clay
- 1-2 oz of Powdered Herbs (see below for suggestions)
- Water or Aloe Vera Juice (enough to make a paste)
- 1-2 drops of Essential Oil added only at time of application

Choose a cosmetic clay (Bentonite clay or even Neem powder, work well).

**Suitable Herbs for this recipe.** Choose according to your skin type. Citrus peel powders (lemon, orange, grapefruit, etc.) add astringency; rose petal powder adds hydration. Both types are great for adding fragrance and anti-bacterial properties. **Feel free to mix and match** your herbs and clays. Other suitable powdered ingredients are milk powder, honey powder, cocoa powder and even powdered or milled oatmeal. All of which can be easily ordered online.

Combine powdered ingredients to make 4 oz of dry clay mixture. Store in a separate container. **Do not** pre-mix or store your dry mixture with your wetting agent.

To use, add approximately ½ oz of the dry clay facial herb blend to a small bowl and mix enough warm water or Aloe Vera juice to make a paste. Add a drop or 2 of essential oil if desired.

Apply mixture in gentle circular motions and allow to dry for about 15-20 minutes. This is the perfect time for you to connect with The Divine energy that is within you and everywhere around you.

When you're done, rinse clean with warm water. Make sure you follow-up with a thorough cleanse or two. Be sure to tone and moisturize well after this oil dissolving mask.

**Variations:** Experiment with other wetting agents. Something like a cucumber puree to cool the skin or strawberry puree to impart alpha-hydroxys. Yogurt is an excellent agent to soften the skin or the lactic acid in milk is good to remove dead cells from the surface of your skin.

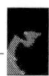

## *Flax Seed Facial*

Flaxseeds are so good for you. Whether you take them internally, or use them topically, you will benefit tremendously from incorporating flaxseeds into your beauty program.

I'm sure you've heard of using flax seed gel on your hair, but flaxseed gel is also fantastic for caring for your skin!

**TO MAKE FLAXSEED GEL:**

Boil ¼ cup of flax seeds in 1 cup of water for 10–20 minutes. Stir constantly. Water will begin to be filled with mucous and foam. Continue to stir. Once gel is desired consistency, strain through sieve, or even stocking. Gel will thicken as it cools.

**VARAIATIONS AND ADDITIONS YOUR SKINCARE:**

You may add things like aloe gel or juice, Vitamin E, Jojoba, Essential Oils etc. Get creative here!

When you've created your perfect blend, apply this mixture to your face, neck and hands. You can use your fingers or a brush for application. A thicker layer (or several paintings) will be more tight and flaky, requiring a rinse; good for PM treatments. A lighter application makes a wearable daytime moisturizer.

These masks and ingredient options will do your skin a world of good, both in the short-term and definitely for your long-term goals. Customize your recipes and use what works best for your skin type, budget and objectives.

## Fruit Salad Facial

This recipe is bursting with alpha-hydroxy acids, nourishing enzymes and healing goodness. Your skin will adore you and others will adore your skin!

Make sure your fruit is very ripe for this recipe!

### Ingredients:

- ½ Banana
- ¼ Avocado
- ¼ Cantaloupe
- 1 Tbsp of Wheat Germ or Wheat Germ oil
- 1 Tbsp of Yogurt
- 1 or 2 Vitamin E capsules or 1 tsp of bulk Vitamin E Oil

Blend ingredients thoroughly into a paste. Apply a thick layer to your skin.

Go listen to some good music for about 15 minutes. Once you're done, rinse clean with warm water. Finish with a few splashes of cold. **This recipe is also a winner for your hair!**

## Banana Cake Face

Blend together ½ of a banana, 1 tablespoon honey, 1 egg yolk, ½ teaspoon almond oil and 1 tablespoon plain yogurt. Honey stimulates and smoothes, yogurt and almond oil penetrate and moisturize and the egg refines and tightens your pores.

This one will be thick, so go dance for about 15 minutes while the mixture works into your skin. When you're feeling really good, come back and rinse clean; first with warm water and then with cold.

Finish with a toner and light moisturizer.

## ~ *Natural Skin Care Conclusion* ~

Build a foundation with sound skincare fundamentals to ensure that your skin remains healthy and radiant. Developing a routine of skincare basics will serve you now and far into the future.

**Just remember the basics:**
- **Cleansing:** Twice daily
- **Toning:** After cleansing
- **Moisturizing:** After toning
- **Exfoliating:** Weekly or Bi-Weekly
- **Masking:** Once or twice per month

It's really very simple and most days, only takes minutes.

Women of Color are blessed with the perfect skin for natural radiance, anti-aging, protection and resilience. Fortifying your skin's natural ability to shine is an act of true Self-Love.

**You deserve to be pampered.**

Chances are you're the one that takes care of everyone else. Make taking care of yourself a priority! Make the space and time to love on your skin and you'll love your skin on you!

**Cultivate your natural beauty by *BEING* beautiful and you will naturally *LOOK* more beautiful!**

For more powerful natural skincare recipes visit Amazon and **download my skincare guide "I Wanna Eat Your Face"**. It's full of cleansers, toners, moisturizers, anti-aging treatments and much more, for ALL skin types!

**Enjoy Enhancing Your Natural Beauty!**

## ~ *About the Author* ~

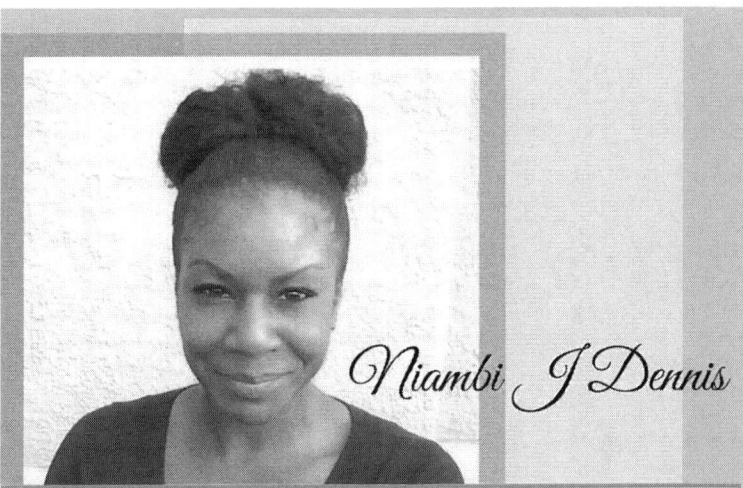

**Niambi J. Dennis is a Licensed Esthetician** and has been a Skincare Consultant for over 6 years. She specializes in natural treatments and remedies for the care and maintenance of healthy skin. She sees clients regularly in her treatment room, providing services and aftercare coaching for vibrant, glowing skin.

Niambi is a former professional athlete, personal fitness trainer, sports development coach, Army recruiter and highly sought after Speaker. Since body health and skin health go hand in hand, she's been able to successfully transfer these skills into a successful Skincare Coaching and Healthy Living practice.

Niambi hosts workshops promoting empowerment, personal development and a healthy living lifestyle. She speaks regularly on various topics ranging from skincare, natural hair care, health & fitness and clean eating.

Please explore her series of Skin Care books all available on Kindle at Amazon.

## ~ *Other Books by This Author* ~

### GROOMING & PERSONAL CARE

**I Wanna Eat Your Face** – 100 Homemade Facial Recipes for Radiant and Ravishing Skin

**Beauty is More than Skin Deep** - Foods & Beverages Teas & Tonics for Enhancing Your Natural Beauty

**Natural Care for Your Ethnic Hair** - Natural Hair Care for Women of Color

**Skin Care Beauty Basics for Women of Color** – Natural Skincare for Beautiful Brown Skin

**Juicy Beauty** – 21 Day Juicing and Smoothie Program for Enhancing Your Natural Beauty

### PERSONAL DEVELOPMENT

**Your Voice is a Force** - Speak to Succeed

### MORE TITLES COMING SOON!!!

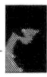

# I invite you to take a look at my complete line of Skin Care & Healthy Living Guides

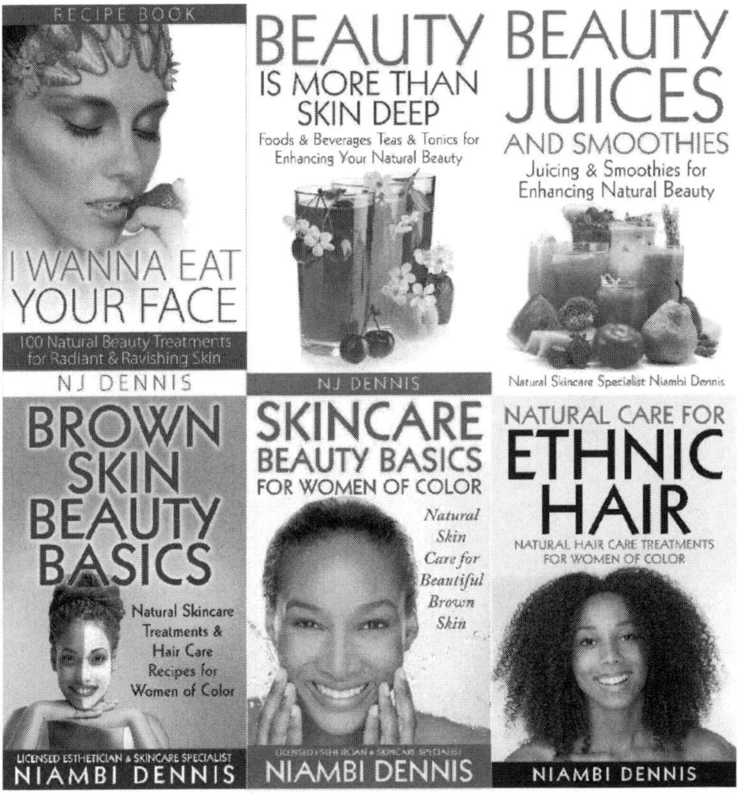

## ~ *One More Thing* ~

Thank you so much for your support and purchasing this book! I hope you have enjoyed the tips and recipes and have found them useful. To empower and to live empowered is my truest intention. I'd like to sincerely thank you for allowing me to live out that intention.

If you have enjoyed this book and will be using these simple and fun recipes to naturally care for your skin, please let me know, by leaving me a quick review!

Your support really means the world to me. I'd be very grateful. Post a short REVIEW for this book through the Amazon order page. I personally read all reviews and use your feedback to make my work even better.

THANKS FOR LEAVING A GREAT REVIEW ON THIS BOOK!

Again, your support is invaluable!

Thank you so sincerely,

**Niambi J Dennis**

*Dedicated to my Dad, Percy Gatewood Dennis, with Love.
I will keep you alive in my heart, for the rest of my days...*

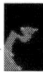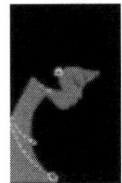

Printed in Great Britain
by Amazon